Ilona Pole
Diana R. Schwartz

The Secrets

OF YOUR

health

Healthy Food Books
New York
2021

Ilona Pole
Diana R. Schwartz
THE SECRETS OF YOUR HEALTH

ISBN 978-1-955001-01-4

Published by
Healthy Food Books
New York, USA
healthyfoodbooks@gmail.com

Book & Cover Design by
Bagriy & Company
Chicago, USA

Sponsored by

A POLE
www.stretchyourspine.com

NutriD
www.nutridbody.com

Printed in United States of America

DISCLAIMER

This book contains the opinions and ideas of its authors. It is intended to provide helpful general information on the subjects that it addresses. It is not in any way a substitute for the advice of the reader's own physician(s) or other medical or health professionals based on, among other things, the reader's own age, weight, gender, current or prior individual conditions, medication history, laboratory data, symptoms, or concerns, and other factors unique to the reader. If the reader needs personal medical, health, dietary, exercise or other assistance or advice, the reader should consult a competent physician and/or other qualified health care professionals. The author and publisher specifically disclaim all responsibility for injury, damage, or loss that the reader may incur as a direct or indirect consequence of following any directions or suggestions given in the book or participating in any programs described in the book, or any other use of this book including without limitation any medical judgments or in connection with any resulting diagnosis and treatments.

The fact that a physician, medical professional, organization, or web site is mentioned in this book, as a potential source of information or treatments, does not mean that the author or the publisher endorses any particular physician or medical professional, or the information they may provide, or the medications, equipment products, or courses of treatment they may have used or recommended.

Contents

The Basis for Good Health

The Detox Diet

Recipes

The Basis of Good Health

Human Immune System

The immune system is a system of biological structures and processes in the body that ensures the body's protection from viruses and infections and other pathogens. It is also responsible for evacuation of toxins and waste out of the body.

When the immune system is weak, the body becomes susceptible to viruses, infections, and parasites.

The immune system is based on the following factors:

> HEALTH is a multi-level (biochemical, psychological, and energetic) balance, i.e., the balanced function of all the systems and organs of the body. The foundation of good health is the immune system, which helps fight off viruses in the body.

- Your lifestyle
- Your mindset
- Your nutrition
- Your physical activity
- Your genetics that form in utero, i. e., your parents' health

Normally, some people only start thinking about their health and immune support when they get sick, which already signifies an immunodeficiency or a weakened immune system.

Immunodeficiency is a state of compromised immune system, which can be reversible or irreversible, caused by various reasons and factors of your life.

The purpose of your immune system is to identify and respond to harmful pathogens, viruses, infections, and parasites by either removing or destroying them.

The immune system consists of the central organs (such as bone marrow and thymus). The immune system closely interacts with other systems: endocrine, nervous, digestive, circulatory, and lymphatic, as well as the organs of the body that contain lymphoid tissue (lymphocytes of various stages of maturity), spleen, lymphatic nodes, Peyer's patches in the intestine, tonsils, and the appendix. Each organ of the immune system performs its specific function.

The Spine — Key
to a Strong Immune System

The condition of your internal organs and your body's systems depends on the condition of the spine. The spine is also the main channel that connects all the organs of the body with the brain. In some cases, the condition of the spine is the cause of the internal organs' dysfunctions. In others, dysfunctions of internal organs can impact various parts of the spine. Disruption of balance in the organs and systems weakens the body's defensive abilities (i. e., immune system).

A POLE was created to maximize the depth and effectiveness of relaxation, to relieve back muscle pain, the lumbar and cervical parts of the spine, abdominal and chest muscles, diaphragm, arms, rib cage, ligaments, and tendons, and to release the sciatic nerve and the spine overall.

> To support a healthy spine,
> we recommend exercise equipment
> called A POLE

Exercising on A POLE allows you to make your spine more flexible in a short time. Decompression and stabilization of the spine with the help of A Pole equipment will help straighten your posture by stretching and lengthening the tense and weak muscles and by eliminating the imbalance and pain. It will reduce muscle tension and pressure on intervertebral discs, increase flexibility of ligaments, and relax and strengthen the muscles and overall ligament systems. The exercises will restore flexibility and movement to muscles, ligaments and tendons, and improve the blood flow in the arteries, veins, and lymphatic systems.

To schedule a consultation, go to:
www.stretchyourspine.com
or call: (929) 334–6060.

Taking care of your body and strengthening your immune system is the foundation of good health, happiness, and success.

The Main Building Blocks
of a Strong Immune System

- Balanced diet
- Healthy sleep
- Physical activity — that helps strengthen your immune system
- Positive thinking

The Main Building Blocks
of a Healthy Balanced Diet

- On an empty stomach, drink warm water (may add lemon).
- Consume natural foods and aim to eliminate processed foods, canned products, foods that contain synthetic dyes, artificial flavors, sugar, sugar substitutes, and yeast.
- Consume fresh fruits and vegetables, whole grains, legumes, and nuts.
- Include fermented vegetables and fruits prepared through the fermentation process (see recipe for fermented fruits and vegetables on page 37).
- In small amounts use: olive oil, avocado oil, mustard oil, cold pressed sesame oil, cold pressed linseed oil, and flaxseed oil.
- Unless you are lactose-intolerant, you can include, in moderation: natural yogurt, kefir, buttermilk, butter, cottage cheese, whole milk cheeses, fresh cream, and sour cream. If you are lactose-intolerant, substitute with almond, soy, or oat milk.
- In moderation (once or twice a week) consume meat such as lamb, veal, beef, rabbit, and alternate it with poultry such as chicken, turkey, or quail.
- Once or twice a week eat fish and other seafood, preferably, wild-caught.
- Try to substitute sugar for honey.

Digestive system issues directly affect your immunity. Overeating, consuming sweet and fatty foods, baked goods, and carbonated beverages lead to various issues that weaken your immune system and, therefore, the ability of your body to resist viruses and harmful bacteria.

The Main Building Blocks
of Healthy Sleep

The most important factor for healthy sleep is a comfortable environment in your bedroom:

- The ideal temperature is 68-71 °F (20-22 °C) with humidity at 50-60 %.
- Air out your bedroom every day.

Additional actions for healthy sleep include:

- Try to go to bed at the same time every night. The best time for bed is before 11 pm. At this time, most people's bodies are ready to relax.
- Two to three hours before bed, eat a light meal (for example, vegetables, fruits, yogurt, or kefir — replace with dairy free options if lactose intolerant).
- Take a walk outdoors before bed.
- A cup of chamomile or mint tea before bed will help you fall asleep faster and easier.
- It is good to take a warm bath or shower before bed.

Healthy sleep is one of the main factors that affect your life expectancy. If you wish to be healthy and live long and happily, you should stick to a schedule, and minimize stress that affects your healthy rest and sleep. A human must sleep as much as predetermined by nature. Everyone has their individual norm that may vary, but on average, an adult needs 7-9 hours of sleep. A person that has had enough sleep is more capable both physically and mentally than someone who slept poorly or not enough.

This is why — It's important to make sure you are getting healthy sleep.

Functions of Healthy Sleep

- Allow your body to rest.
- Allow your organs and systems to recharge to support normal function.
- Restore your immunity.

Sleep and rest affect your immune system and lack thereof weakens your immune response to infection, viruses, and elimination of toxins.

Hormones in your body function as immunomodulators that regulate the sensitivity of your immune system.

Depression and stress lead to the release of corticosterone and cortisol, and these, along with an imbalance of hormonal activity, suppress your immune system and, as a result, increase your immunodeficiency.

The Main Principles
of Physical Activity for Strengthening
Your Immune System

- Regular daily or 2-3 times a week of exercise.
- Gradual increase in physical activity.

The Basis of Good Health

Once you decide to improve your health, start exercising slowly and at a minimal level. Once you feel comfortable with the activity level, gradually increase the intensity.

▪ • Adequately pick the type of physical activity.

When choosing your physical activity, follow your preferences (walking, bicycling, swimming, etc.) and account for your physical shape, the state of your spine, and your daily schedule.

> Physical activity has to be both healthy and fun!

Lack of *physical activity* can lead to an imbalance in the body. When the amount of calories consumed exceeds the amount of energy burned off, the metabolism slows down. The slower the metabolic system, the less caloric intake is required. The excess calories will translate into fat which can lead to lymphatic system not working properly. The lymphatic system is responsible for eliminating waste, acids, and toxins out of your body.

> Overly vigorous exercise, i.e., overworking your body, can lead to acidosis in the body.

Overworking is a state of the body when it cannot recover quickly after physical, psychological, or emotional strain. Symptoms of overworking include fatigue, anxiety, elevated heart rate, insomnia, irritability, low immunity, and frequent colds.

The Importance
of Your Body's Acid-Base Balance

The balance between acids and bases in your body is called the pH level and it should stay between 7 and 7.5 (ranging from 0 being the most acidic to 14 being the most basic). Having an acid-base imbalance towards acidic pH is called acidosis and can lead to organ dysfunction and illness. For balanced function of your internal organs, the pH level should be greater than 7, indicating a slightly basic (alkaline) level.

> The healthiest drink is alkaline water!

The acid-base balance is the gauge of health. The more "acidic" we are, the faster we get sick and the faster we age.

Maintaining the acid-base balance in the body promotes strengthening of the immune system and overall health.

Water is a liquid that creates suitable conditions for biochemical processes in your body.

Alkaline water is the healthiest option with the pH level of 7.5 or greater.

Water plays a vital role in the functions of the body and actively participates in almost every vital process. For instance, when water enters the body, it provides nutrients to cells and cleanses them from waste.

> Healthy ("alkaline") foods—fresh vegetables, fruits, greens, sprouted grains and legumes.

The filtration and excretory systems of your body — the lymph, sweat, and urine — are liquids in which the eliminated waste is dissolved.

In an "acidic pH" body, the cells are deprived of oxygen and nutrients. The acid-base imbalance makes your body susceptible to disease and can cause sickness and health issues. The body will attempt to compensate for the acidic pH with base minerals. If the diet does not contain sufficient minerals to compensate, acids accumulate in the body's fat and other tissues.

The main way to strengthen your immune system is to enrich your diet with green foods that contain chlorophyll. Chlorophyll brings oxygen to your cells and, therefore, speeds up your metabolism and eliminates toxins from your body. Green and white vegetables and fruits will help you remain healthy, beautiful, and slim. The main attributes of vegetables and fruits is their high content of chlorophyll, fiber, and phytochemicals, all of which positively affect your digestive system and metabolism. Vegetables and fruits help cleanse your intestinal wall. When consuming vegetables and fruits, you lessen the strain on your digestive system, your kidneys and liver. Your body will have an easier job of eliminating toxic waste in a natural manner.

> Acidic foods include: baked goods, sugar, sugar substitutes, coffee, meat, carbonated drinks, processed foods, canned foods, yeast, marinades, vinegar, mayonnaise, and margarine.

It is recommended that you consume 80 % alkaline and 20 % acidic foods, although some dietitians may shift this to 60/40 %.

The Detox Diet

The Detox Diet may improve the function of your digestive system and strengthen your immunity.

The Detox Diet is a *temporary* change in the diet. It functions to naturally eliminate wastes and toxins from the body, and helps to restore vital functions and energy in a short period of time.

The Main Goals of the Detox Diet

- Strengthen the body's defensive abilities
- Balance and regulate digestion
- Improve metabolism
- Improve kidney function, eliminate excessive fluid and swelling
- Eliminate toxins and waste from the body
- Normalize body weight
- Reduce the severity of allergies
- Improve condition of the skin on the face and body
- Improve overall well-being
- Improve energy levels

The Main Rules of the Detox Diet

It is important to prepare for the detox diet in advance by entering it gradually and without stress on the body.

Several days (3-5 days) prior to starting the detox diet, you should decrease consumption of fried food, salty food, dairy, yeast, baked goods, bread, sugar, coffee, red meat, and fatty fish.

Try to substitute with vegetables, fruits, mushrooms, legumes, and grains.

A diet is a temporary process to normalize your bodily functions

Food	Substitute
Butter, margarine	Olive oil, avocado oil, coconut and other plant oils
Canned fruit and vegetables	Fresh or frozen fruits and vegetables
Coffee	Herbal and fruit tea
Sugar	Raw honey, stevia
Red meat	Poultry (chicken, quail, turkey), rabbit
Milk, cream	Almond milk, flaxseed milk, oat milk
Carbonated drinks	Fresh fruit and vegetable juices, smoothies, lemon water
White potatoes	Sweet potato, yuca, taro
White rice	Brown and wild rice
Bread containing yeast	Yeast-free bread

Start your morning with a glass of warm or room temperature water (can add lemon, if tolerable), this helps with awakening the digestive system. Stick to your personal meal schedule. do not overeat, take small frequent meals, and eat dinner 2-3 hours before bed.

The diet is based on a certain temporary limitation of food consumption and substituting meals with healthier options.

To start the detox diet, first pick days for the detox diet that are most convenient for you. If possible, do not plan to follow the detox diet during the time of intensive physical activity. It is beneficial to combine the detox diet with walks, biking, swimming, massage, physical therapy, exercise, and moderate physical activity. This will increase the detox's effectiveness.

Remember that the detox diet does not mean you should be fasting. You do not have to suffer and feel uncomfortable. Moderation is the key.

Create and stick to a meal schedule that works best for you, which should include 4-6 meals a day with small portions.

During the detox diet, drink approximately ½ gal (1.5L-2L) of water a day (preferably alkaline water). This will help eliminate toxins out of your body and speed up your metabolism. There are detox diets of various lengths, and if you find limiting your meals difficult, start with more basic and shorter-period options.

For detox diet beginners, start with a 1-3 day detox. Once you successfully achieved the three-day detox, move on to a seven-day detox diet. In the future, progress to a more advanced level of 14 days or longer.

The main rules are: "do no harm" and "everything in moderation".

A detox diet is not recommended for pregnant and nursing women, children, teenagers, the elderly, as well as for people with heart conditions, chronic conditions, diabetes, and those with low blood sugar levels.

The detox diet is primarily based on consuming green vegetables and fruits, sprouted grains, and whole grains. To make the detox diet more effective, you have to eliminate: sugar, yeast, baked goods, dairy, eggs, meat, fish, caviar, seafood, salty/spicy/fried/smoked foods, pre-made condiments, mayonnaise, canned foods, coffee, cocoa, sweet carbonated drinks, spices, pickled and marinated foods.

> Before you start the detox diet,
> talk to your health care provider!

If you do not have a registered dietitian nutritionist, our offices can help. To schedule a consultation, go to: www.NutriDbody.com or call: 347–394–4995.

During the detox diet the food preparation will be based on boiling, stewing, steaming, sautéing or baking.

In the post-detox diet phase, food should be reintroduced just as gradually as the pre-detox diet phase. The transition period of post and pre-detox diet phases is about three days. During that time, you are reintroducing foods back in limited amounts.

The Detox Diet below is an example, which you can change based on your needs and goals.

Sample Menu for DD-Diet #1

You can adjust meals yourself, from a period of one to up to seven days, based on your preferences and goals, swapping meals based on the list of ingredients or substituting foods that suit you.

On an empty stomach: warm water (can add lemon).

Breakfast: steel cut oatmeal cooked in water (can add fruit).

Snack: salad, Russian vinaigrette (boiled beets, potatoes, carrots, cucumbers, green onions, and olive oil).

Lunch: brussels sprouts soup (onion, turnip, carrot, brussels sprouts, green bell pepper, potato, parsley, dill, garlic, and olive oil).

Snack: carrot muffins.

Dinner: salad (stewed or baked fennels, parsley, garlic, and olive oil). Buckwheat.

On an empty stomach: warm water (can add lemon).

Breakfast: apple muffins.

Snack: boiled rice and sautéed spinach with onions.

Lunch: pumpkin soup (Butternut squash).

Snack: baked apples.

Dinner: vegetable stew (onion, bell pepper, zucchini, carrot, potato, and olive oil), cucumber salad.

Su	Mo	Tu	We	Th	Fr	Sa
			1	2	3	4
5	6	7	8	9	10	11
12	13	14	15	16	17	18
19	20	21	22	23	24	25
26	27	28	29	30		

Su	Mo	Tu	We	Th	Fr	Sa
			1	2	3	4
5	6	7	8	9	10	11
12	13	14	15	16	17	18
19	20	21	22	23	24	25
26	27	28	29	30		

On an empty stomach: warm water (can add lemon).

Breakfast: quinoa with green vegetables.

Snack: pumpkin muffins.

Lunch: asparagus soup (asparagus, onion, German turnip, green bell pepper, carrot, parsley, potato, and olive oil).

Snack: fruit.

Dinner: grilled or baked vegetables (onion, bell pepper, squash), mashed potatoes.

On an empty stomach: warm water (can add lemon).

Breakfast: amaranth porridge (cooked in water) with stewed apples.

Snack: sautéed vegetables (zucchini, onion, carrot, bell pepper, root celery, and olive oil), mashed peas.

Lunch: spinach soup (taro, spinach, bell pepper, onion, carrot, parsley, and olive oil).

Su	Mo	Tu	We	Th	Fr	Sa
				1	2	3	4
5	6	7	8	9	10	11
12	13	14	15	16	17	18
19	20	21	22	23	24	25
26	27	28	29	30		

Snack: lemon cookies.

Dinner: stuffed baked squash (boiled rice, stewed squash, carrot, onion, eggplant, olive oil).

On an empty stomach: warm water (can add lemon).

Breakfast: pumpkin with rice.

Su	Mo	Tu	We	Th	Fr	Sa
				1	2	3	4
5	6	7	8	9	10	11
12	13	14	15	16	17	18
19	20	21	22	23	24	25
26	27	28	29	30		

Snack: buckwheat with a salad (avocado oil, onion, cucumber, Napa cabbage, parsley, dill, avocado, lemon).

Lunch: borscht (cabbage, beetroot and beet greens, bell pepper, onion, carrot, garlic, potato, parsley, dill, oil, lemon).

Snack: fruit or a smoothie.

Dinner: salad (cucumber, leeks, lemon, olive oil, arugula, spinach, parsley and other greens), boiled yuca.

On an empty stomach: warm water (can add lemon).

Breakfast: oatmeal with fruit.

Su	Mo	Tu	We	Th	Fr	Sa
			1	2	3	4
5	6	7	8	9	10	11
12	13	14	15	16	17	18
19	20	21	22	23	24	25
26	27	28	29	30		

Snack: oat milk pudding with banana and chia seeds.

Lunch: cream of onion soup with taro (oil, white onion, carrot, taro, bell pepper, parsley).

Snack: banana muffins.

Dinner: baked vegetables (oil, onion, bell pepper, asparagus, potato, cactus, lemon).

Su	Mo	Tu	We	Th	Fr	Sa
			1	2	3	4
5	6	7	8	9	10	11
12	13	14	15	16	17	18
19	20	21	22	23	24	25
26	27	28	29	30		

On an empty stomach: warm water (can add lemon).

Breakfast: millet cereal.

Snack: green salad (boiled root celery, bell pepper, parsley, cucumber, green onion, boiled potato, oil, lemon).

Lunch: mint soup (carrot, oil, chives, spinach, mint, parsley root, dill, bell pepper, green onion, potato).

Snack: apple baskets.

Dinner: artichoke hearts with vegetables (artichoke, onion, carrot, sweet peas, potato, oil, lemon, parsley).

Sample Menu for DD-Diet #2
(Green Ingredients Only)

You can adjust meals yourself, from a period of one to up to seven days, based on your preferences and goals, swapping meals based on the list of ingredients or substituting foods that suit you.

Sprouts (wheat or buckwheat sprouts can be added to salads or have by itself throughout the day)

On an empty stomach: warm water (can add lemon).

Breakfast: whole grain oats cooked in water.

Snack: salad (boiled root celery, green bell pepper, parsley, cucumber, green onion, boiled potato, dill, oil, lemon, avocado).

Su	Mo	Tu	We	Th	Fr	Sa
				1	2	3	4
5	6	7	8	9	10	11
12	13	14	15	16	17	18
19	20	21	22	23	24	25
26	27	28	29	30		

Lunch: vegetable soup with green beans (oil, onion, German turnip, green beans, green bell pepper, parsley, dill).

Snack: kiwi fruit.

Dinner: vegetable salad (cucumber, leek, arugula, spinach, parsley, lemon, olive oil). Buckwheat.

The Detox Diet

On an empty stomach: warm water (can add lemon).

Breakfast: apple muffins.

Snack: boiled rice, green salad, avocado.

Su	Mo	Tu	We	Th	Fr	Sa
			1	2	3	4
5	6	7	8	9	10	11
12	13	14	15	16	17	18
19	20	21	22	23	24	25
26	27	28	29	30		

Lunch: lentil soup (oil, onion, green bell pepper, turnip, green lentils, parsley).

Snack: baked apples.

Dinner: grilled vegetable stew (oil, onion, zucchini, bell pepper, potato), salad (arugula, spinach, onion, avocado, lemon, olive oil).

On an empty stomach: warm water (can add lemon).

Breakfast: cream of buckwheat.

Snack: lemon cookies.

Lunch: asparagus soup (oil, onion, German turnip, green bell pepper, asparagus, potato, parsley, garlic).

Su	Mo	Tu	We	Th	Fr	Sa
			1	2	3	4
5	6	7	8	9	10	11
12	13	14	15	16	17	18
19	20	21	22	23	24	25
26	27	28	29	30		

Snack: fruit (kiwi, apple).

Dinner: grilled vegetables (onion, bell pepper, asparagus, brussels sprouts, zucchini, lemon), boiled yuca.

On an empty stomach: warm water (can add lemon).

Breakfast: amaranth porridge.

Snack: green salad (boiled celery root, green bell pepper, cucumber, boiled potato, green onion, parsley, dill, oil).

Su	Mo	Tu	We	Th	Fr	Sa
				1	2	3	4
5	6	7	8	9	10	11
12	13	14	15	16	17	18
19	20	21	22	23	24	25
26	27	28	29	30		

Lunch: sorrel soup (onion, turnip, green bell pepper, potato, sorrel, parsley, dill, olive oil).

Snack: fresh-pressed apple juice.

Dinner: steamed vegetables (broccoli, bell pepper, celery stalks), boiled rice.

On an empty stomach: warm water (can add lemon).

Su	Mo	Tu	We	Th	Fr	Sa
				1	2	3	4
5	6	7	8	9	10	11
12	13	14	15	16	17	18
19	20	21	22	23	24	25
26	27	28	29	30		

Breakfast: muffin.

Snack: buckwheat, avocado (guacamole).

Lunch: broccoli soup (onion, turnip, green bell pepper, potato, broccoli, parsley, garlic, dill, olive oil).

Snack: fresh-pressed celery juice.

Dinner: vegetable salad (cucumber, onion, arugula, spinach, avocado, parsley, avocado oil, lemon). Mashed peas.

On an empty stomach: warm water (can add lemon).

Breakfast: whole oats.

Snack: quinoa salad (cucumber, green onion, bell pepper, avocado, boiled quinoa).

Lunch: cream of taro soup (oil, onion, green bell pepper, turnip, taro, parsley, spinach).

Snack: pear.

Dinner: baked vegetables (oil, yuca, onion, green bell pepper, broccoli, asparagus).

Su	Mo	Tu	We	Th	Fr	Sa
			1	2	3	4
5	6	7	8	9	10	11
12	13	14	15	16	17	18
19	20	21	22	23	24	25
26	27	28	29	30		

On an empty stomach: warm water (can add lemon).

Breakfast: bulgur (cooked in water).

Snack: salad (celery stalks, green bell pepper, cucumber, parsley, green onion, dill, avocado, oil, lemon), buckwheat.

Lunch: pea soup (oil, green peas, onion, turnip, green bell pepper, parsley).

Su	Mo	Tu	We	Th	Fr	Sa
			1	2	3	4
5	6	7	8	9	10	11
12	13	14	15	16	17	18
19	20	21	22	23	24	25
26	27	28	29	30		

Snack: fresh-pressed apple juice.

Dinner: sautéed fennels with onion (oil, fennels, onion, parsley), boiled rice.

Dysfunctions of the Digestive System

There are various types of diets: Protein, Atkins, Ketogenic, Dukan, mono-diets, etc. Your nutritionist will suggest an individual diet for your particular needs and goals.

DD-Diet #3 suits those with digestive tract issues, IBS, Crohn's disease, and ulcerative colitis.

Issues with the gastrointestinal (GI) tract, such as IBS, Crohn's disease, and ulcerative colitis can tell us right away that there is inflammation present in the GI system. The main goal is to reduce inflammation with healthy gut-nutrition and exclude products that inflame, irritate, or damage the GI tract.

It is also necessary to clear the bowel lining of mucus and old compacted fecal matter, and parasites which may also cause inflammation and irritation.

You may possibly need an anti-parasitic regimen. Consult your doctor and registered dietitian nutritionist.

> *If you do not have a registered dietitian nutritionist, our offices can help. To schedule a consultation, go to: www.nutridbody.com or call: 347–394–4995.*

Moderate nutrition, combined with cleansing of your digestive system and gastrointestinal system, is the basis for treating digestive disorders.

The Main Dietary Principles
for Irritable Bowel Syndrome (IBS),
Crohn's Disease, and Ulcerative Colitis

- Eat small meals every two to three hours.
- Drink 8 cups of water a day (preferably alkaline water).
- Wash fruits and vegetables well and peel them.
- Eat stewed, sautéed, steamed, or boiled fruit and vegetables (do not fry!).
- Use olive or mustard oil, or cold pressed linseed oil (in small amounts).
- Include oatmeal, buckwheat, pearl barley, quinoa, wild and brown rice.
- Drink water 20 minutes before or 30 minutes after a meal.

Sample Menu for DD-Diet #3
(Green Ingredients Only)

Avoid:

- Meat and poultry.
- Fish, seafood, shellfish.
- Dairy (milk, buttermilk, yogurt, cheese, butter).
- Salted, pickled, marinated foods.
- Dried fruit.
- Nuts.
- Honey.

- Baked goods.
- Yellow and red vegetables and fruits.
- Legumes.
- Cabbages (white cabbage, broccoli, turnip, brussels sprouts, Napa cabbage, radish, all vegetables in cabbage family).
- Watermelon, cantaloupe, pears, grapes, raisins.
- Canned juices.
- Canned foods.

> Eliminate all types of cabbage.
> Completely eliminate
> SALT, SUGAR, SPICY FOOD, SPICES.
> Note: to eliminate sugar, we recommend substituting toothpaste (which contains sugar) for baking soda with lemon.

Recommended:

- Grains: rice, buckwheat, oat, bulgur, quinoa.
- Olive oil and other plant oils.

> The main principle of nutrition for IBS is consuming steamed, stewed, or boiled fruits and vegetables.

- Green vegetables: scallions, white onions, leeks, green bell pepper, squash, zucchini, avocado, celery, spinach, cucumbers, asparagus, artichoke, potatoes, yuca, parsley, greens, dill, sorrel, arugula, cactus, mint, aloe, and celery root.
- Green fruits: apples, kiwi, gooseberry, lemon.

You can adjust meals yourself, from a period of one to up to seven days, based on your preferences and goals, swapping meals based on the list of ingredients or substituting foods that suit you.

On an empty stomach: warm water.

Breakfast: rice porridge cooked in water.

Snack: cookies.

Lunch: vegetable soup (onion, celery root, celery, green bell pepper, potato, parsley root, parsley, dill, and olive oil).

Su	Mo	Tu	We	Th	Fr	Sa
			1	2	3	4
5	6	7	8	9	10	11
12	13	14	15	16	17	18
19	20	21	22	23	24	25
26	27	28	29	30		

Snack: baked apples.

Dinner: vegetable stir fry (onion, zucchini, bell pepper, potato, and olive oil).

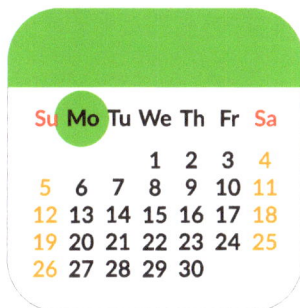

On an empty stomach: warm water.

Breakfast: oatmeal.

Snack: potato stew (potatoes, onion, asparagus, bell pepper).

Lunch: zucchini soup (rice, onion, celery root, green bell pepper, zucchini, parsley root, parsley, dill, olive oil).

Su	Mo	Tu	We	Th	Fr	Sa
			1	2	3	4
5	6	7	8	9	10	11
12	13	14	15	16	17	18
19	20	21	22	23	24	25
26	27	28	29	30		

Snack: stewed green apples.

Dinner: baked asparagus, buckwheat.

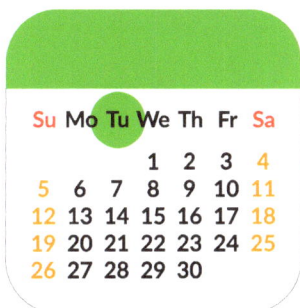

On an empty stomach: warm water.

Breakfast: whole grain oat cooked in water.

Su	Mo	Tu	We	Th	Fr	Sa
			1	2	3	4
5	6	7	8	9	10	11
12	13	14	15	16	17	18
19	20	21	22	23	24	25
26	27	28	29	30		

Snack: cooked rice with sautéed spinach and onions.

Lunch: asparagus soup (onion, celery root, asparagus, green bell pepper, parsley root, parsley, potato, olive oil).

Snack: gooseberry compote (do not add sugar).

Dinner: grilled vegetables (onion, bell pepper, zucchini, cactus). Mashed potatoes.

On an empty stomach: warm water.

Breakfast: amaranth porridge.

Snack: cookies.

Su	Mo	Tu	We	Th	Fr	Sa
			1	2	3	4
5	6	7	8	9	10	11
12	13	14	15	16	17	18
19	20	21	22	23	24	25
26	27	28	29	30		

Lunch: cream of celery soup (onion, green bell pepper, potato, celery, celery root, parsley root, parsley, dill, olive oil).

Snack: stewed apple baskets.

Dinner: grilled zucchini with parsley, dill. Mashed potatoes.

On an empty stomach: warm water.

Breakfast: barley porridge.

Snack: green salad (boiled celery root, green bell pepper (peeled), peeled cucumbers, green onions, boiled potato, dill, oil).

Su	Mo	Tu	We	Th	Fr	Sa
			1	2	3	4
5	6	7	8	9	10	11
12	13	14	15	16	17	18
19	20	21	22	23	24	25
26	27	28	29	30		

Lunch: green vegetable soup (onion, celery root, potato, green bell pepper, beet-greens, parsley root, parsley, dill, olive oil).

Snack: cookies.

Dinner: quinoa salad with mixed greens.

On an empty stomach: warm water.

Breakfast: oatmeal.

Snack: grilled zucchini, buckwheat.

Lunch: cream of taro soup (onion, green bell pepper, taro, parsley root, parsley, olive oil).

Su	Mo	Tu	We	Th	Fr	Sa
			1	2	3	4
5	6	7	8	9	10	11
12	13	14	15	16	17	18
19	20	21	22	23	24	25
26	27	28	29	30		

Snack: baked apples.

Dinner: baked vegetables (yuca, onion, green bell pepper, asparagus, cactus, squash, olive oil).

On an empty stomach: warm water.

Breakfast: steel-cut oats.

Snack: cookies.

Su	Mo	Tu	We	Th	Fr	Sa
				1	2	3	4
5	6	7	8	9	10	11
12	13	14	15	16	17	18
19	20	21	22	23	24	25
26	27	28	29	30		

Lunch: cream of onion soup (oil, onion, green bell pepper, taro, celery root, celery).

Snack: fresh-pressed apple juice.

Dinner: sautéed fennel with onions (fennels, parsley, dill, lemon). Boiled rice.

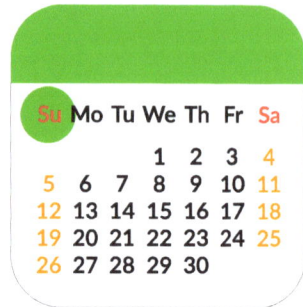

These are fairly simple diets, but it does not mean that you must strictly stick to them. We showed you an example of easily accomplishing the goal of fixing your digestion and immunity by selecting healthy meals. You can change the meal plan based on your individual needs and capabilities.

These diets are for educational and recommendation purposes, but they are not personalized. If you have any questions, contact your doctor or registered dietitian nutritionist (RDN).

If you do not have a registered dietitian nutritionist, our offices can help. To schedule a consultation, go to: www.nutridbody.com or call: 347–394–4995.

You will be helped by Diana R. Schwartz, RDN, LD, CDN.

RECIPES

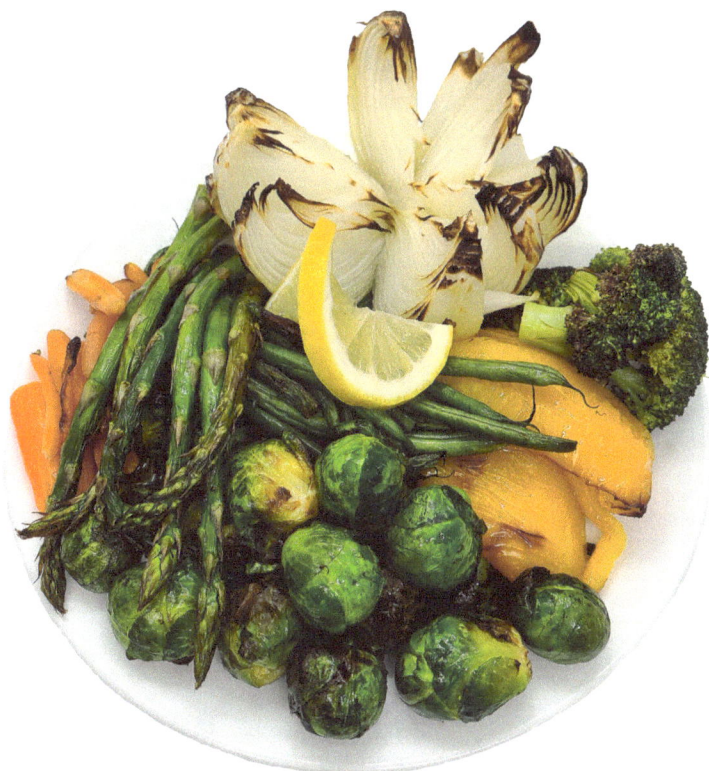

Buckwheat

1 cup buckwheat, 2 ½ cups water, bring to boil, then simmer on low heat for 15-20 min, until water is absorbed.

Rice

1 cup rice, 1 ½ cups water, bring to boil, then simmer on low heat for 15-20 min, until water is absorbed.

Steel-cut Oats

1 cup oats, 5 cups water, bring to boil, then simmer on low heat for 20-30 min until water is absorbed (soak oats in water overnight; without soaking oats overnight, steel-cut oats will cook for about 2 hours).

Whole Grain Oats

5 tbsp oats, 2 cups water, bring to boil, then simmer on low heat while stirring for 3-5 min.

Millet

1 cup millet, 3 cups water, bring to boil, cover it, and then simmer on low heat for 20-30 min.

Pearl Barley

1 cup barley, 2 cups water, bring to boil, cover it, and then simmer on low heat for 40-60 min.

Introduction to Fermented
Fruits and Vegetables

Fermentation: a process to preserve fruits and veggies that also increase healthy bacteria. Great replacement for pickling!

Fermented foods are made by lacto-fermentation. Lacto-fermentation is a process where bacteria breakdown sugars in fruits and veggies to form lactic acid.

Lactic acid preserves the food from spoiling and enriches it with vitamins B, K, C, Omega-3 fatty acids, and various probiotics.

Fermented foods also provide prebiotics, which feed probiotics and can lead to increased healthy gut bacteria in the body.

Fermented foods support your body's flora. These beneficial bacteria are powerful detoxicators that can eliminate toxins and heavy metals out of your body. Fermented foods are healthy for people with diabetes since they improve pancreatic function.

Fermented products can also improve peristalsis, pancreas, and gallbladder functions as well as stimulate digestive juices for digestion. They also act as powerful natural biologically active supplements.

Sauerkraut

Ingredients:
- 1 small head of cabbage
- 1 medium carrot
- 2 tbsp salt (rock or Himalayan)
- 3 tbsp honey

Prepare approximately 1 gallon (3 liter) jar. Slice the cabbage thinly. Grate the carrot.

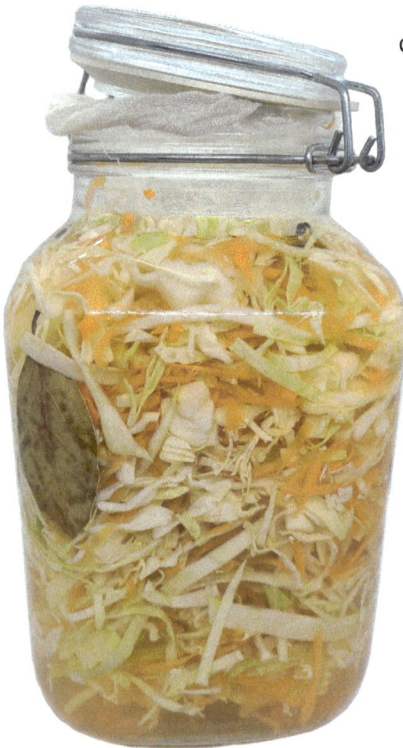

Combine cabbage and carrot. Put in the jar loosely, leaving the top 2 in. (5 cm) empty. Pour cold water in, to the top of the jar.

Cover with cheese cloth, touching the water. Put salt in the cheesecloth, cover with a plate and put in a dark place for 24 hours.

Remove the cheesecloth, add honey. Cover with a plate and leave in a dark place for another 48 hours.

Cabbage is ready to eat after 72 hours. Keep refrigerated.

vegetables and fruits

Fermented Cucumbers

Ingredients:
- 8-10 small cucumbers
- a head of garlic
- dill
- 1 tsp mustard seed
- 1 tsp cilantro seed
- 1-2 bay leaves
- celery stalk (optional)

Brine:
- 2 tbsp rock or pink Himalayan salt per 1 quart (1 liter) of water.

For the brine, pour water into a pot, dissolve salt in it.

Wash cucumbers thoroughly and place in the jar.

Separate garlic cloves, peel, wash, and place in the jar with spices.

Pour in the brine to cover the contents, cover with a plate, and store in a cool dark place for five days. Murky brine is okay.

Cucumbers will be ready in 120 hours. Keep refrigerated.

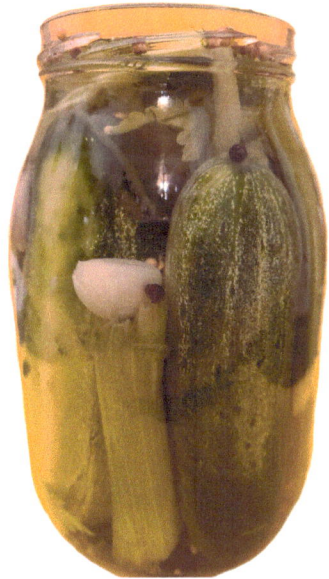

Fermented Apples

Ingredients:

- 3-4 medium apples
- 1 cinnamon stick
- 2 tbsp salt (rock or Himalayan)
- 1 quart (1 liter) of water
- 1 tbsp honey

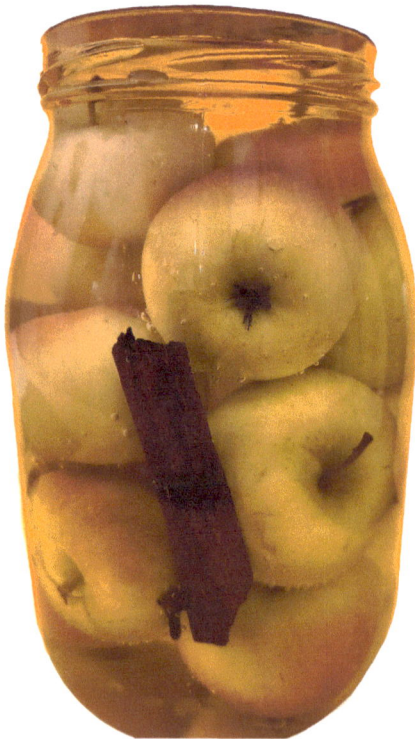

Thoroughly wash the apples, cut in half and place in a quart-size jar.

Pour water in a pot, add salt and cinnamon, bring to a boil. Let cool.

Pour the brine into the jar. Add honey.

Cover with a plastic lid and store in a dark place for 5-7 days.

Keep refrigerated.

vegetables and fruits

Fermented Assorted Vegetables

Ingredients:
- 1 head cauliflower, separated into florets
- 1 head of garlic
- 1 lb. tomatoes
- dill
- 1 tsp mustard seed
- 1 tsp cilantro seed
- 1-2 bay leaves
- 1 celery stalk (optional)

Brine:
- 2 tbsp rock or pink Himalayan salt per 1 quart (1 liter) of water.

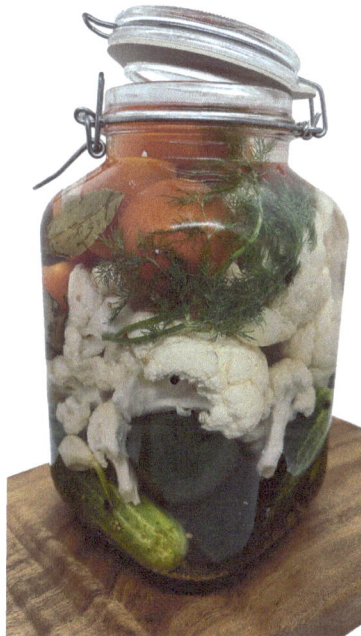

Pour 2 quarts (2 liters) of water in a pot, dissolve 4 tbsp salt. Do not boil.

Wash vegetables thoroughly and place in layers in a 1-gallon (3 liters) jar.

Separate garlic cloves, peel, wash and place in the jar with spices.

Pour brine into the jar to cover the contents. Cover with a plate.

Put in a cool dark place for five days. Murky brine is okay.

Keep refrigerated.

Brussels Sprouts Soup

Ingredients:
- 10 brussels sprouts
- 1 green bell pepper
- 1 head of German turnip
- 2-3 potatoes
- 1 onion
- celery root
- celery
- dill
- 3 garlic cloves
- lemon
- bay leaf
- 2 tbsp oil or canola oil

Cut vegetables into small cubes.

Put cut onion, German turnip, celery root, bell pepper into a pot. Add oil, bay leaf, and garlic.

Cover with 2 cups of water and stew for 15-20 min covered on low heat until halfway cooked.

When vegetables are soft, add potatoes and brussels sprouts. Add 1-1.5 quarts (1-1.5 liters) of boiled water. Cook until brussels sprouts and potatoes are done. Add parsley and dill.

Add salt and other spices to taste based on your goals.

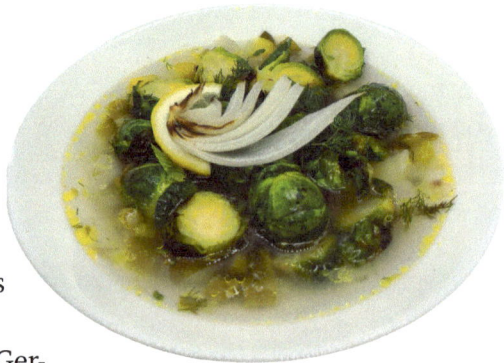

soups

Asparagus Soup

Ingredients:
- 1 onion
- 1 german turnip
- 1 green bell pepper
- a bunch of asparagus
- 3 potatoes
- parsley root
- parsley
- dill
- bay leaf
- 3 garlic cloves
- 2 tbsp oil or canola oil

Cut vegetables into small cubes.

Put cut onion, German turnip, parsley root, bell pepper and asparagus into a pot. Add oil and garlic.

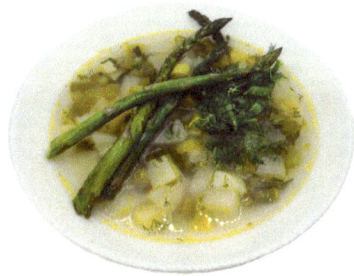

Cover with 2 cups of water and stew for 15-20 min covered on low heat until halfway cooked.

When vegetables are soft, add cubed potatoes. Add 1-1.5 quarts (1-1.5 liters) of boiled water. Cook until potatoes are done. Add parsley and dill.

Cooking time is approximately 40 minutes.

Add salt and other spices to taste based on your goals.

Broccoli Soup

Ingredients:

- 1 onion
- 1 german turnip
- 1 head of broccoli
- 1 green bell pepper
- 3 potatoes
- parsley root
- parsley
- dill
- 3 garlic cloves
- bay leaf
- 2 tbsp oil or canola oil

Cut vegetables into small cubes.

Place cut up onion, German turnip, parsley root, bell pepper and asparagus into a pot. Add oil, bay leaf and garlic.

Cover with 2 cups of water and stew for 15-20 min covered on low heat until halfway cooked.

When vegetables are soft, add cubed potatoes. Add 1-1.5 quarts (1-1.5 liters) of boiled water. When potatoes are done, add broccoli separated into small florets, parsley, and dill. Cook for another 3 min.

Add salt and other spices to taste based on your goals.

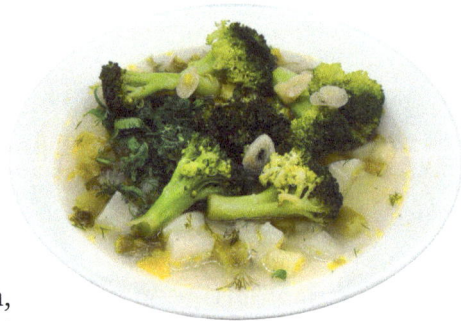

soups

Cream of Taro Soup

Ingredients:
- 1 german turnip
- 2 onions
- a medium taro (1 lb.)
- 1 green bell pepper
- parsley root
- parsley
- dill
- 3 garlic cloves
- bay leaf
- 2 tbsp olive oil or canola oil

Cut vegetables into small cubes.

Put cut onion, German turnip, parsley root and bell pepper into a pot. Add oil, bay leaf, and garlic.

Cover with 2 cups of water and stew for 15-20 min covered on low heat until halfway cooked.

When vegetables are soft, add taro. Add 1.5 quarts (1.5 liters) of boiled water. Cook until taro is done. Add parsley and dill and take bay leaf out. Let the soup cool a little and cream in a blender.

Add salt and other spices to taste based on your goals.

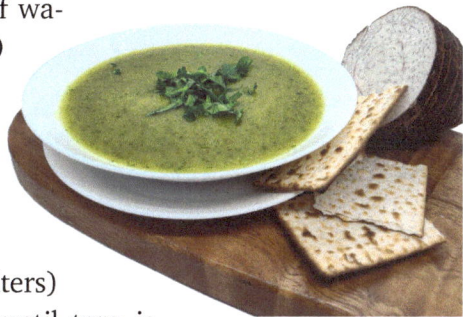

Green Bean Soup

Ingredients:

- 1 german turnip
- 2 onions
- a bag of green beans (1 lb.)
- 1 green bell pepper
- parsley root
- parsley
- dill
- 3 garlic cloves
- bay leaf
- 2 tbsp oil or canola oil

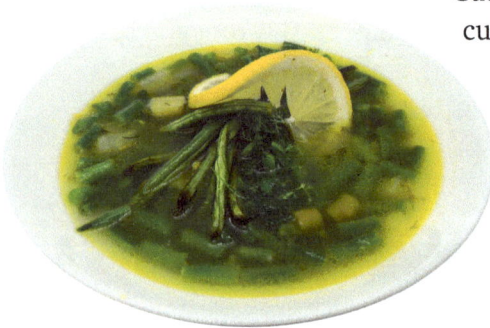

Cut vegetables into small cubes.

Place cut up onion, German turnip, parsley root and bell pepper into a pot. Add oil, bay leaf, and garlic. Cover with 2 cups of water and stew for 10 min covered on low heat until halfway cooked.

Add green beans, cut in 1-inch pieces. Add 1-1.5 quarts (1-1.5 liters) of boiled water. Cook until green beans are done. Add parsley and dill.

Add salt and other spices to taste based on your goals.

appetizers
and salads

Baked Vegetables

Ingredients:
- 1 onion
- 1 head of broccoli (separated into florets)
- 2 bell peppers
- 2-3 potatoes
- 1 zucchini
- celery stalks
- bay leaf
- 2-3 tbsps. olive oil

Preheat the oven to 350 °F.

Cut vegetables and mix in a bowl with oil. Place into a baking pan and add a cup of water. Cover with aluminum foil and bake for 40 min at 350 °F.

Baking time may vary depending on your oven. Monitor the process.

Add salt and other spices to taste based on your goals.

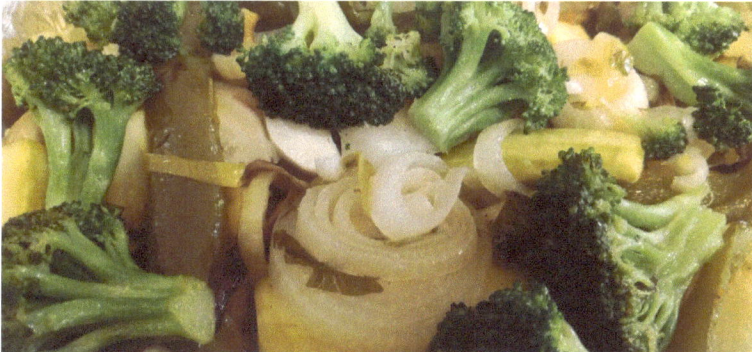

Healthy Potato Pancakes

Ingredients:

- 1 onion
- 2 potatoes
- a handful of spinach
- 3-4 tbsp oat flour
- 1 tbsp olive or canola oil
- ½ tsp baking soda slaked with lemon juice

Grate potatoes and onion finely into a bowl. Add oat flour, oil, slaked baking soda and finely chopped spinach. Mix well.

Line a baking sheet with parchment paper.

With a tablespoon, put small circles of the mixture on the paper. Press each circle down lightly.

Bake at 350 °F. Flip pancakes after 5 min and bake for additional 5 min.

Baking time may vary depending on your oven. Monitor the process.

Add salt and other spices to taste based on your goals.

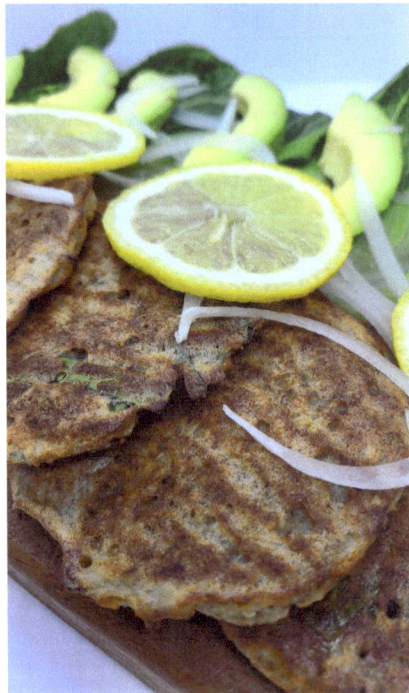

appetizers and salads

Green Salad

Ingredients:
- 1 bunch of green onions
- ½ celery root
- 1 green bell pepper
- 3 cucumbers
- 1 yuca (or 2-3 potatoes)
- parsley
- dill
- 1 lemon
- olive oil

Cook celery root and yuca (or potatoes) and let cool.

Cube vegetables. Combine all ingredients, add parsley and dill, lemon juice and olive oil.

Add salt and other spices to taste based on your goals.

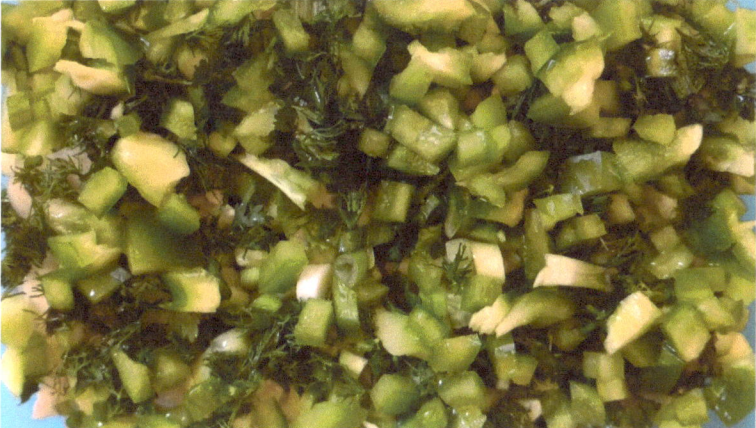

Oatmeal and Chia Seed Pudding

Ingredients:

- 4 tbsp oatmeal
- 1 pint water
- 1 large ripe banana
- 3 tbsp chia seed
- 1 tbsp honey (optional)

Soak oatmeal in cold boiled water for 15 min. Mix in a blender with banana, add honey (optional).

Pour into a bowl, add chia, mix.

Put mixture in cups.

Leave for 1 hour to let chia rise.

Ready in 1 hour.

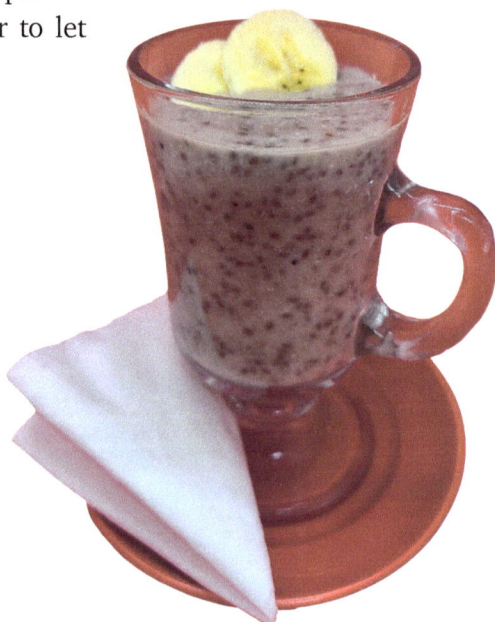

desserts

Quick Oatmeal

Ingredients:
- 2 cups water
- 5 tbsp quick oats
- 1 tbsp oil

Heat water in a pot. Do not boil. Slowly add oats, mixing in with a whisk to avoid clumping. Cook 2-3 min from the start of boiling on low heat.

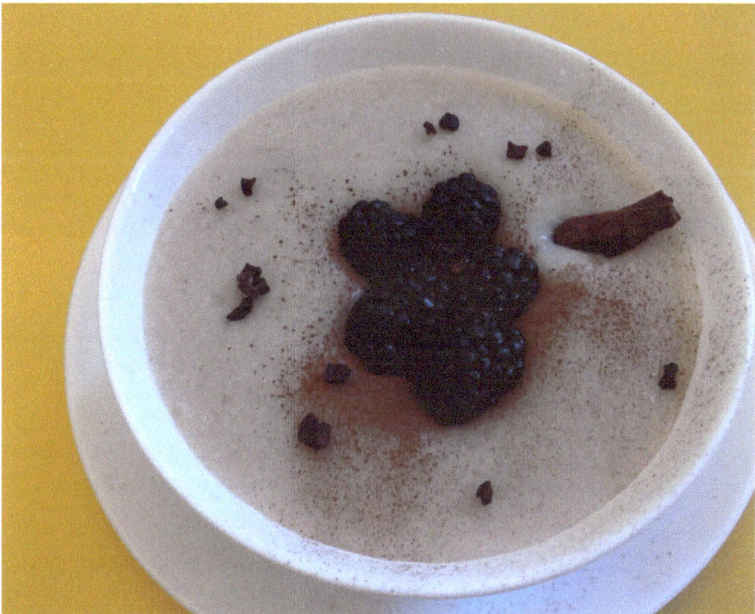

Banana and Chocolate Muffins

Ingredients:
- 2 tbsp oats
- 1 cup oat flour
- 1 cup water
- 2 bananas
- ½ cup corn flour
- 2 tbsp oil
- 2 tsp cocoa powder
- ½ tsp baking soda
- ½ lemon

Make a cup of oat milk: mix 2 tbsp oat flour with 1 cup water and let stand 15 min.

Mix in a blender with bananas. Pour mixture in a bowl. Add ground oats and corn flour. Slake baking soda with lemon juice. Add oil. Mix ingredients together.

Divide in two parts. Add cocoa to one part.

Put batter into 12 paper muffin cups or one larger baking dish, oiled. Alternate the two mixtures, creating layers.

Bake 15-20 min at 350 °F.

Baking time may vary depending on your oven. Monitor the process.

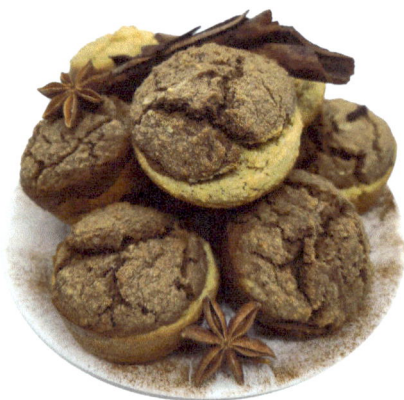

desserts

Pumpkin Cookies

Ingredients:

- 7 oz (200 g) pumpkin
- 10.5 oz (300 g) oat flour
- 3 tbsp oil or canola oil
- ½ tsp baking soda
- 2 lemons
- ½ tsp cinnamon (optional)
- honey

Finely grate pumpkin. Add oat flour and finely grated lemon zest. Add baking soda, 3 tbsp lemon juice, oil, and cinnamon. Mix thoroughly.

To avoid dough sticking to hands, wet hands with water.

Form small balls. Put onto a baking sheet covered in parchment paper. Number of cookies will depend on the size of the balls.

Bake for 15-20 min at 350 °F. Baking time may vary depending on your oven. Monitor the process.

Let cookies cool. Eat with honey, if desired.

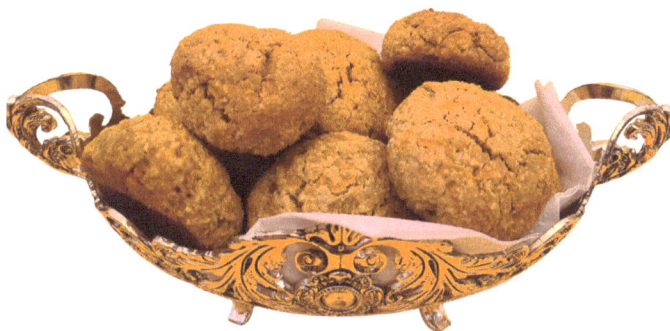

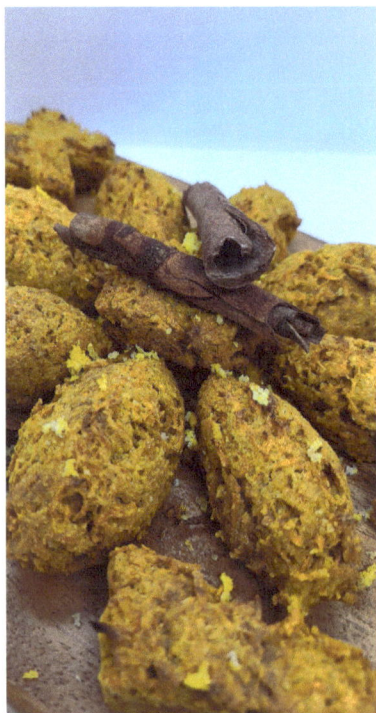

desserts

Carrot Cookies

Ingredients:
- 2 medium carrots (1 lb.)
- 1 cup oat flour
- 1 cup semolina flour
- 3 tbsp coconut oil
- 1 tsp baking soda
- 2 lemons
- 1 tsp cinnamon
- 2 tbsp honey

Finely grate carrots. Add semolina flour, oat flour and finely grated zest of two lemons. Slake baking soda with juice of one lemon. Add coconut oil, honey, and cinnamon.

Mix all ingredients and let stand 10-15 min to let batter rise.

To avoid dough sticking to hands, wet hands with water.

Shape dough into small balls. Place onto a baking sheet covered in parchment paper. Number of cookies will depend on the size of the balls.

Bake for 15-20 min at 350 °F. Baking time may vary depending on your oven. Monitor the process.

Let cookies cool. Eat with honey, if desired.

desserts

Apple Cookies

Ingredients:
- 2 large green apples
- 2 cups oat flour
- 2 heaping tbsp semolina flour
- 2 tbsp oil
- ½ tsp baking soda
- 1 lemon
- honey

Grate apples on medium grater. Add oat flour, semolina flour, finely grated lemon zest, oil and baking soda. slaked with lemon juice.

Mix all ingredients. Let stand 10-15 min to allow batter to rise. Density of dough will depend on the juiciness of apples. If dough is runny, add oat flour. Dough should be soft and form easily. Shape dough into small balls and press down lightly. To avoid dough sticking to hands, wet hands with water.

Place balls onto a baking sheet covered in parchment paper. Number of cookies will depend on the size of the balls.

Bake for 15-20 min at 350 °F. Baking time may vary depending on your oven. Monitor the process.

Let cookies cool. Eat with honey, if desired.

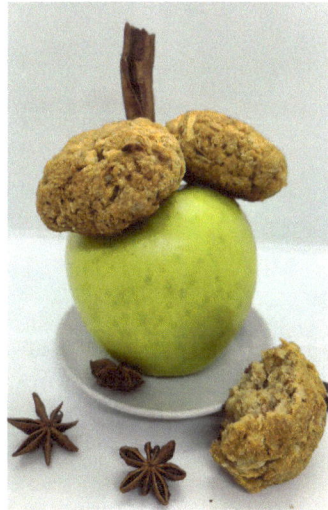

Stewed Apple Baskets

Ingredients:

- 1 cup oat flour
- 1 cup corn flour
- 2 tbsp oil or canola oil
- ½ tsp baking soda
- 1 lemon
- ½ cup water
- 2 green apples for filling

In a bowl, mix oat and corn flours and finely grated lemon zest. Add oil, water, and baking soda slaked with lemon juice.

Mix the ingredients. The dough should be soft and easy to shape.

Shape dough into small balls and flatten tops slightly. Place in a baking pan lined with paper baking cups. Lightly

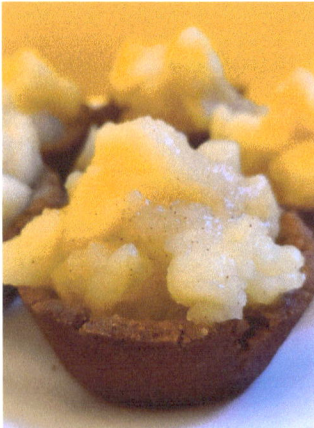

wet your hands with water to avoid sticking and shape dough pieces into baskets. Bake 10 min at 350 °F. Baking time may vary depending on your oven. Monitor the process.

Cut apples into small cubes and place in a small pot. Add 2 tbsp water. Stew covered 3 min. Add cinnamon (optional). Let cool. Place filling into baskets before eating.

desserts

Lemon Cookies

Ingredients:
- 2 lemons
- 1 cup oat flour
- ¾ cup semolina flour
- 3 tbsp (coconut) oil
- ½ tsp baking soda
- 1 tbsp honey

Grate lemon zest into a bowl. Add 2 oz lemon juice, baking soda, honey, and oil.

Add semolina flour. Let stand 10 min to allow semolina to rise.

Add ¾ of oat flour saving the rest for rolling dough.

Mix dough. It should be soft and easy to roll and shape. Shape dough into small cookies, place on a baking sheet covered with parchment paper. Number of cookies will depend on their size.

Bake 10 min at 350 °F. Baking time may vary depending on your oven. Monitor the process.

Let cool before eating. Add honey, if desired.

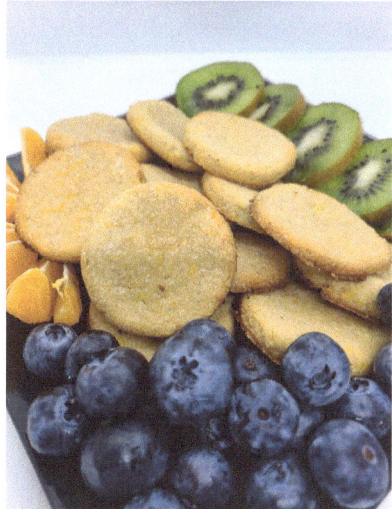

desserts

Banana Cookies

Ingredients:
- 1 cup almond milk
- 2 bananas
- 1 cup oat flour
- 1 cup semolina flour
- 1 tbsp coconut oil
- ½ tsp baking soda
- ½ lemon

Almond Milk Recipe: Soak 1 cup of almonds in warm water. 20 min later, peel off the skin of the almonds. Place the peeled almonds into a blander with 1 cup of water, blend well. Pour the blended mixture through a cheesecloth. Almond milk is ready.

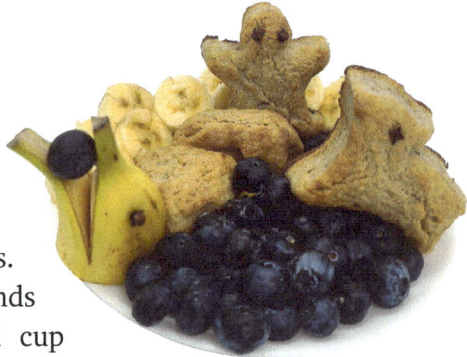

Add mashed bananas, oat flour, semolina flour, coconut oil, and baking soda slaked with lemon juice, in with the almond milk. Mix well.

Place mixture into a muffin pan lined with paper muffin cups (or oiled, if no paper cups). You should have 12 cookies.

Bake 10 min at 350 °F. Baking time may vary depending on your oven. Monitor the process.

NUTRI
D

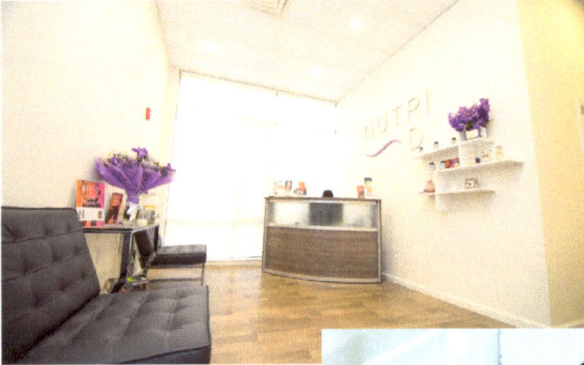

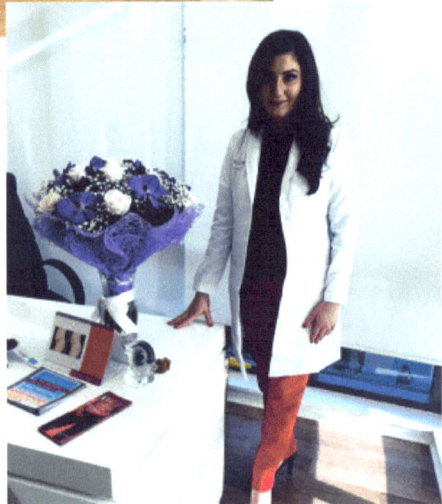

Diana R. Schwartz,
RDN, LD, CDN

Registered Dietitian Nutritionist
(347) 394–4995

Like us on Facebook: Facebook.com/NutriDBody
Follow us on Instagram: @NutriDbody
www.nutridbody.com

A POLE

www.stretchyourspine.com

To support a healthy spine, we recommend exercise equipment called A POLE

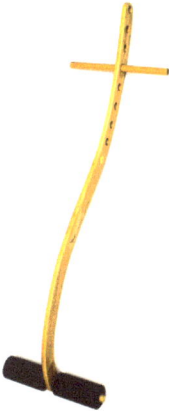

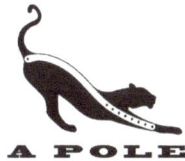

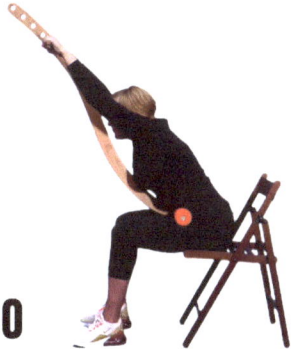

www.ingramcontent.com/pod-product-compliance
Lightning Source LLC
Chambersburg PA
CBHW040125270326
41926CB00001B/24